The Calm Bladder Code

Rewire Your Body, Reclaim Your Health, and Break the UTI Loop

BRENDA HARCOURT

Copyright

Contents

DISCLAIMER

This book is intended for informational purposes only. The author and publisher do not guarantee specific outcomes from the methods, strategies, or recommendations discussed. While the content is based on research and patient experiences, individual results may vary.

This book is not a substitute for professional medical advice, diagnosis, or treatment. Readers should consult a qualified healthcare provider before making any changes to their diet, lifestyle, or treatment plan.

Every effort has been made to ensure the accuracy and relevance of the information presented. However, the author and publisher are not responsible for any errors, omissions, or outdated content. Personal anecdotes included in this book are based on real experiences, though names and identifying details may have been altered to protect privacy.

By applying the insights and recommendations in this book, readers acknowledge and accept full responsibility for their health decisions

Introduction

Welcome to Freedom from Recurrent UTIs

Living with a Urinary Tract Infection (UTI) is far more than just a series of uncomfortable physical symptoms. It's a cycle that robs you of your peace, your sense of control, and at times, even your confidence. If you're reading this, you might already know the frustration that comes with frequent doctor visits, rounds of antibiotics, and a feeling of powerlessness over your own health. Perhaps you've tried cranberry juice, countless pain relievers, or even over-the-counter remedies with little success—and worse, you've found yourself battling yet another infection just when you thought it was over.

But what if I told you that you don't have to live this way?

This book is not about quick fixes, masking symptoms, or offering you a simple solution that will leave you feeling unsatisfied and unhealed. Instead, **The Empowered UTI Solution** is about something deeper. It's about **holistic**

healing, long-term prevention, and empowering you to take control of your health. Here, you'll find the support, practical tools, and knowledge you need to understand and tackle the root causes of UTIs—and the emotional, physical, and mental toll they take on you.

Rather than just treating the symptoms, we're going to **transform the way you approach your UTI experience**. From mindset shifts to preventive habits, from medical insights to self-care strategies, you'll uncover what truly works and why certain common treatments often fall short.

If you're ready to stop feeling like a victim to your body's struggles and start taking an active role in your healing journey, keep reading.

Chapter 1

Understanding the Primary Complaint: The Burden of UTIs

Unpacking the Emotional, Physical, and Mental Toll

Urinary Tract Infections (UTIs) are often dismissed as a minor, temporary inconvenience. But for many, these infections are more than just a simple medical issue—they represent a profound and often overwhelming burden on daily life. While the physical symptoms of a UTI are hard to ignore—burning sensations during urination, pelvic pain, and the constant urge to go—there is a much deeper impact that extends far beyond the body.

The physical discomfort is just the beginning. For those suffering from recurrent UTIs, the emotional toll can be staggering. The sense of urgency to constantly manage symptoms, the fear of the infection spreading, and the frustration of not feeling fully healed, even after treatments, contribute to a heightened sense of anxiety and stress. The unpredictability of the condition—never knowing when the next flare-up will occur—adds an additional layer of emotional exhaustion. It is not just the pain that patients endure, but the mental strain of living with something that feels constant, out of their control, and unrelenting.

Furthermore, the psychological impact cannot be overstated. Many people with recurrent UTIs experience significant feelings of isolation, shame, and frustration. The physical symptoms are often misunderstood by others, leading to feelings of being "invisible" or dismissed by those who can't fully grasp the depth of the problem. For example, in social settings, the fear of an impending UTI attack may cause people to cancel plans, avoid intimacy, or hold back from engaging in activities that would otherwise bring joy. Over time, this sense of isolation can erode a person's confidence, contribute to depression, and trigger feelings of hopelessness. The struggle to manage the infection becomes intertwined with a deeper emotional toll, affecting not only their mental health but also their relationships and quality of life.

In our approach to treating UTIs, it is vital to recognize the complexity of the issue. It's not just a "bladder infection" but an ongoing emotional, physical, and mental battle. This chapter aims to lay the groundwork for understanding that UTI management cannot be confined to just eradicating bacteria; it must also address the entire person—their body, mind, and spirit.

Why Traditional Solutions Fall Short

It's no secret that the conventional medical approach to UTIs relies heavily on antibiotics. When an infection arises, the first response is often to prescribe antibiotics to kill the bacteria responsible. While this can offer immediate relief, it fails to address the bigger picture. Antibiotics may eradicate the infection temporarily, but they don't offer a sustainable solution for those suffering from recurring UTIs. The underlying causes—such as hydration, hygiene, stress, or anatomical factors—are often overlooked.

Moreover, the overuse of antibiotics is not without its consequences. Antibiotic resistance is an ever-growing concern, meaning that recurrent infections might become more difficult to treat with each successive round of antibiotics. This creates a cycle of dependency on medications that are not always effective in the long term, and in some cases, the infection may not be fully eradicated, leading to persistent or recurring issues. This cycle leads to frustration and a sense of helplessness, as many patients feel they are merely "managing" the infection rather than eliminating it for good.

Traditional treatments like cranberry supplements and over-the-counter urinary pain relief medications also fail to provide lasting solutions. While cranberry juice and pills are often touted as a natural remedy for UTIs, scientific evidence supporting their effectiveness remains limited. They might offer minor benefits, like preventing bacteria from adhering to the urinary tract, but they cannot address active infections or prevent future recurrences. Similarly, urinary pain relief medications only mask the symptoms of a UTI without addressing the root cause, meaning the infection continues to simmer beneath the surface, setting the stage for the next flare-up.

Even with these short-term fixes, the emotional and mental burden remains unaddressed. The stress, anxiety, and fear associated with UTIs often go unnoticed or unspoken. These treatments focus on the infection itself, but fail to heal the emotional scars caused by recurrent flare-ups, leaving many patients feeling disempowered and alone in their struggle.

The Invisible Struggles

While the physical symptoms of a UTI are undeniable, it is the invisible struggles that truly shape a patient's life. The emotional impact of recurrent UTIs often goes unacknowledged in medical discussions, but it is no less important.

Chronic pain and discomfort are not the only burdens; feelings of shame, fear, and anxiety take a significant toll on mental health. The stress of anticipating a UTI at any moment can cause a person to constantly feel on edge, leading to heightened levels of anxiety. The unpredictability of when the next flare-up might occur can cause individuals to withdraw from social interactions or avoid physical intimacy, further deepening feelings of isolation.

The constant vigilance required to manage UTIs can also lead to burnout. Whether it's constantly drinking water, taking supplements, or adhering to hygiene rituals, the mental load can feel endless. For many patients, this mental burden is as exhausting, if not more so, than the physical symptoms. The pressure to always "do the right thing" in order to prevent another infection can feel overwhelming, and the constant sense of failure when an infection occurs despite efforts to prevent it adds to feelings of inadequacy.

Additionally, there is the sense of frustration when others do not understand the depth of the condition. UTIs are often dismissed as "just a bladder infection," leading to misunderstandings from family, friends, and even healthcare providers. This lack of empathy can be deeply isolating, leaving individuals to feel as though their struggles are invalid or unimportant. The emotional toll of feeling misunderstood or dismissed can make the healing process much harder.

To make matters worse, many individuals with UTIs experience ongoing feelings of guilt or self-blame. They may wonder if they could have done more to prevent the infection or if their lifestyle choices were to blame. These negative thought patterns only serve to intensify the emotional burden and prevent them from truly healing.

The invisible struggles of UTIs are real, and they deserve to be addressed in any comprehensive treatment plan. As we progress through this book, we will provide practical tools for addressing both the physical and emotional aspects of living with recurrent UTIs. By recognizing and validating these invisible struggles, we can begin to heal on a deeper level, moving toward a life free from the constant cycle of infections.

Chapter 2

The Holistic Approach to Healing

Beyond Antibiotics

For many individuals suffering from recurrent urinary tract infections (UTIs), antibiotics are often the go-to solution. While these medications can provide temporary relief by eliminating the bacteria causing the infection, they fail to address the underlying issues that contribute to recurrence. In fact, over-reliance on antibiotics can lead to antibiotic resistance, making future infections harder to treat and creating a vicious cycle that many people feel trapped in.

The problem with antibiotics lies not just in their temporary effectiveness but in their singular focus on eradicating the infection without considering the broader health picture. Antibiotics do nothing to address the lifestyle factors that may be contributing to UTIs, nor do they offer a sustainable solution for preventing future flare-ups. This is where a holistic approach comes into play—one that takes into account the physical, emotional, and mental health of the individual and provides lasting solutions that go beyond simply treating the infection.

A holistic approach views health as an interconnected system, recognizing that physical ailments like UTIs don't occur in isolation. Instead, they are influenced by a wide array of factors such as emotional well-being, stress, diet, and lifestyle choices. By addressing these root causes and making lasting lifestyle changes, individuals can not only prevent future UTIs but also enhance their overall quality of life.

Holistic healing focuses on the whole person, and this chapter will show you how to incorporate lifestyle changes, natural remedies, and emotional resilience techniques to build a strong foundation for long-term health and wellness.

Mind-Body Connection

One of the core elements of a holistic approach to healing is understanding the profound connection between emotional health, stress, and recurring infections. It's easy to think of UTIs as purely physical issues, but stress and emotional imbalances can play a pivotal role in their recurrence.

The relationship between the mind and body is intricate, with emotional stress manifesting in various physical symptoms. When we experience stress, our immune system can become compromised, making us more susceptible to infections. For example, chronic stress or anxiety can reduce the body's ability to fight off bacteria effectively, leaving the urinary tract vulnerable to infections. Stress also impacts our lifestyle choices, leading to habits such as poor diet, inadequate hydration, and insufficient rest—all of which can contribute to the development of UTIs.

Additionally, emotional distress plays a significant role in how we manage our physical health. If we are feeling anxious or overwhelmed, we may neglect self-care practices like hydration or proper hygiene, which are critical in preventing UTIs. Furthermore, the emotional toll of recurrent UTIs—feelings of shame, frustration, and fear of recurrence—can create a cycle of negative emotions that contribute to both physical and mental exhaustion.

By acknowledging the mind-body connection, we can break this cycle. Techniques such as meditation, deep breathing, and mindfulness practices can help to alleviate stress, reduce anxiety, and promote emotional healing. Engaging in these practices helps to restore balance to the nervous system, allowing the body to better manage and ward off infections. Yoga, for instance, can improve circulation and strengthen the pelvic muscles, which are crucial in preventing UTIs, while also calming the mind. The emotional healing achieved through these practices can help create a healthier internal environment, supporting the body's immune function and preventing the recurrence of infections.

A New Way to Heal

The key to sustainable healing from recurrent UTIs lies in making lifestyle changes that address both the physical and emotional aspects of the condition. Rather than relying solely on antibiotics, adopting a holistic approach incorporates a combination of natural remedies, diet, emotional resilience techniques, and self-care strategies. This new way to heal encourages individuals to take an active role in their well-being, shifting away from short-term fixes and focusing on long-term prevention and health optimization.

Lifestyle Changes

To prevent UTIs, lifestyle changes play a crucial role. One of the most important changes is improving hydration. Staying well-hydrated helps to flush bacteria from the urinary tract before it has a chance to cause an infection. Aim to drink plenty of water throughout the day—at least eight glasses—while reducing the intake of sugary or caffeinated beverages that can irritate the bladder.

Another important change is improving hygiene practices. Proper wiping techniques, such as wiping from front to back, and avoiding irritants like harsh soaps or feminine hygiene products, can reduce the risk of bacteria entering the urinary tract. Wearing breathable cotton underwear and avoiding tight-fitting clothes can also help maintain a healthy balance in the genital area.

Nutrition and Supplements

What you eat plays a significant role in your body's ability to prevent and fight infections. A diet rich in antioxidants, vitamins, and minerals can strengthen your immune system, helping your body fight off infections before they can take hold. Specific nutrients, like vitamin C, can acidify urine, which helps prevent bacteria from adhering to the walls of the urinary tract. Incorporating more fruits, vegetables, and whole grains into your diet can provide the necessary nutrients to support your immune system.

Additionally, certain natural supplements, such as cranberry extract and probiotics, can play a supportive role in preventing UTIs. Cranberry has long been thought to help prevent bacteria from adhering to the urinary tract, although scientific evidence remains mixed. Probiotics, on the other hand, help maintain a healthy balance of bacteria in the gut, which can prevent harmful bacteria from entering the urinary tract.

Emotional Resilience

As mentioned earlier, emotional health plays a key role in physical health. Developing emotional resilience through practices such as mindfulness, guided journaling, and emotional healing exercises can help you process the frustration, fear, and isolation that often accompany recurrent UTIs. When we take time to address our emotional well-being, we are better equipped to handle stress and anxiety, which in turn supports our physical health.

One exercise that can be particularly helpful is guided journaling. Writing about your experiences, fears, and frustrations can provide an outlet for emotions that may otherwise go unexpressed. By giving yourself permission to feel and release these emotions, you create space for healing. This simple practice can also help you track patterns in your emotional and physical health, offering insights into potential triggers for recurrent infections.

Interactive Tools and Resources

This book provides a variety of practical tools to help you on your healing journey. You will find symptom trackers to monitor your progress, self-assessments to evaluate your emotional and physical well-being, and personalized action plans that empower you to take control of your health. These tools are designed to support your holistic healing process, ensuring that you are actively engaged in creating lasting change.

Additionally, we offer a directory of online resources, support groups, and specialists who can provide further guidance and emotional support. Reaching out to a community that understands your struggles can provide a sense of solidarity and validation, helping you feel less alone in your journey.

Chapter 3

Preventing Recurrent UTIs: The Power of Lifestyle Change

Urinary tract infections (UTIs) are among the most common health issues affecting millions of individuals, and for those who experience recurrent infections, the cycle can feel endless. While antibiotics may offer temporary relief, they don't address the root causes of these recurring infections. The good news is that simple lifestyle changes can dramatically reduce both the frequency and severity of UTIs. By focusing on hydration, diet, hygiene, and a few natural supplements, you can take control of your health and start healing in a sustainable way.

In this chapter, we'll explore the key lifestyle changes that can prevent UTIs from taking over your life. We'll look at how small shifts in hydration, nutrition, and hygiene can make a big difference, and we'll dive into the role of probiotics and natural supplements in maintaining a healthy urinary system. By adopting a holistic approach to prevention, you'll empower yourself to break the cycle of recurring UTIs and enjoy lasting health.

Hydration, Diet, and Hygiene

The first and most foundational step in preventing recurrent UTIs is adopting healthy habits in hydration, diet, and hygiene. Each of these factors plays a critical role in maintaining a healthy urinary tract, and when they are optimized, the chances of bacterial growth and infection significantly decrease.

Hydration

One of the easiest and most effective ways to prevent UTIs is by ensuring you stay properly hydrated. Drinking plenty of water helps flush bacteria out of your urinary system before it has a chance to take hold. When you are well-hydrated, your body produces more urine, which helps to clear out harmful bacteria from the urinary tract. Aim to drink at least eight glasses of water a day, or more if you are physically active, in hot climates, or if you suffer from conditions like diabetes or kidney disease that may cause dehydration.

Water is the best option for hydration, but certain herbal teas or electrolyte-infused water can also contribute to your hydration levels. However, avoid sugary drinks, sodas, or excessive caffeine, as these can irritate the bladder and increase the risk of infection.

Diet

A balanced diet rich in whole foods—fruits, vegetables, lean proteins, and whole grains— helps support your immune system and keeps your urinary system functioning optimally. Specific foods can also help prevent UTIs by promoting a healthy balance of bacteria in the urinary tract. For example, cranberries have long been recommended for urinary health due to their ability to prevent bacteria from adhering to the bladder walls. While research is still ongoing, many individuals report that drinking unsweetened cranberry juice or taking cranberry supplements has helped them reduce the frequency of infections.

It's also important to focus on foods that promote general immune health, such as foods rich in antioxidants, vitamin C, and probiotics. Citrus fruits like oranges, grapefruits, and lemons are excellent sources of vitamin C, which can acidify urine and inhibit bacterial growth. Additionally, incorporating foods like yogurt and kefir, which contain beneficial probiotics, can help maintain a healthy balance of good bacteria in the urinary tract, making it harder for harmful bacteria to take hold.

Hygiene
Good hygiene is essential in preventing UTIs, as it reduces the likelihood of bacteria entering the urinary tract. Always wipe from front to back after using the bathroom to avoid transferring bacteria from the anal area to the urethra. This simple step can significantly reduce the chances of bacteria entering the urinary system.

Additionally, be mindful of the personal hygiene products you use. Avoid douches, scented wipes, or harsh soaps, as these can irritate the sensitive skin around the genital area and upset the natural bacterial balance. Opt for gentle, fragrance-free products to avoid unnecessary irritation.

When it comes to clothing, choose loose-fitting cotton underwear and avoid tight clothing that may cause moisture buildup, creating an ideal environment for bacteria to thrive. Similarly, make sure to change out of wet clothing, like swimsuits or exercise gear, promptly after sweating, as prolonged moisture can contribute to bacterial growth.

Mindful Eating: Foods That Promote Bladder Health

Your diet plays a significant role in the health of your urinary system. The foods you choose can either support your bladder or cause irritation that may lead to infection. Understanding which foods promote bladder health and which ones should be avoided is crucial in reducing the frequency of UTIs.

Foods to Promote Bladder Health

Certain foods can help support bladder health and reduce the risk of UTIs. As mentioned earlier, cranberries are one of the most commonly recommended foods for bladder health. They contain compounds that prevent harmful bacteria from adhering to the bladder walls, making it more difficult for an infection to take root. Additionally, high-fiber foods such as whole grains, legumes, and vegetables can help improve digestion and overall gut health, which indirectly supports the urinary system.

Probiotic-rich foods like yogurt, kefir, kimchi, and sauerkraut are also beneficial for urinary health. Probiotics help restore the balance of good bacteria in your gut and urinary tract, preventing the overgrowth of harmful bacteria that can lead to UTIs.

Foods to Avoid

Certain foods can irritate the bladder, potentially leading to discomfort or even increasing the likelihood of a UTI. These foods should be limited or avoided if you are prone to recurrent infections:

- **Caffeine**: Found in coffee, tea, and certain sodas, caffeine is a bladder irritant that can increase the frequency of urination and lead to bladder discomfort.

- **Alcohol**: Like caffeine, alcohol can irritate the bladder and disrupt the body's natural processes for flushing out bacteria.

- **Spicy Foods**: Spicy foods can also irritate the bladder and cause discomfort, especially if you have a sensitive urinary system.

- **Artificial Sweeteners**: These can disrupt the balance of bacteria in the urinary tract and lead to irritation.

By focusing on a diet that includes bladder-friendly foods and avoiding irritants, you can significantly reduce your risk of future UTIs and support your body's natural defenses.

The Role of Probiotics and Natural Supplements

In addition to maintaining a healthy diet, certain natural supplements can further support bladder health and reduce the risk of recurrent UTIs. Probiotics and other natural supplements play a pivotal role in maintaining a healthy balance of bacteria in the urinary system.

Probiotics

Probiotics are beneficial bacteria that help restore balance in your gut and urinary tract. These beneficial bacteria can outcompete harmful bacteria, preventing them from colonizing the urinary tract and causing infections. Regularly consuming probiotics, either through food or supplements, can support overall urinary health. Look for supplements that contain strains like *Lactobacillus* and *Bifidobacterium*, as these are particularly helpful for maintaining a healthy microbiome in the urinary system.

Natural Supplements

In addition to probiotics, other natural supplements can help prevent UTIs. Cranberry extract is one of the most well-known supplements for urinary health. It may help prevent bacteria from adhering to the bladder walls, reducing the risk of infection. However, cranberry should be used as part of a broader lifestyle plan, as it is not a cure for an active infection.

Another helpful supplement is D-mannose, a type of sugar found in certain fruits, particularly cranberries, that has been shown to prevent bacteria from sticking to the walls of the urinary tract. Some studies suggest that taking D-mannose as a supplement may help reduce the recurrence of UTIs, particularly in individuals who are prone to recurrent infections.

Herbal Remedies
Certain herbs may also help support bladder health. For example, uva ursi, also known as bearberry, is an herb traditionally used to treat urinary tract infections. It contains compounds that may help reduce inflammation and support the urinary tract. However, it should only be used under the guidance of a healthcare professional, as it may not be suitable for everyone.

By adopting simple lifestyle changes—such as staying hydrated, eating a bladder-friendly diet, practicing good hygiene, and incorporating probiotics and natural supplements—you can significantly reduce the frequency and severity of recurrent UTIs. These changes, combined with a holistic approach to emotional and physical health, can empower you to take control of your health and enjoy a life free from the constant worry of infections.

Chapter 4

The Antibiotics Dilemma: Why They're Not the Ultimate Answer

Antibiotics have long been considered the go-to solution for treating urinary tract infections (UTIs). They can provide quick relief and eliminate the bacteria causing the infection. However, the overuse and misuse of antibiotics have created a growing problem—antibiotic resistance—that threatens both individual health and global well-being. In this chapter, we will explore why antibiotics are not always the ultimate answer for recurrent UTIs, why overreliance on them can be harmful, and what you can do to break free from the cycle of dependence on these drugs.

Understanding Antibiotic Resistance

Antibiotics have revolutionized medicine and saved countless lives since their discovery. Yet, their overuse and misuse have led to a major public health crisis: antibiotic resistance. This occurs when bacteria evolve and become resistant to the drugs that once killed them. As a result, infections that were once easily treatable with antibiotics are becoming harder to manage, leading to longer hospital stays, more complicated treatments, and increased risk of complications.

In the context of UTIs, antibiotic resistance can be particularly problematic. With each course of antibiotics, there is a risk that the bacteria causing the infection will evolve and become resistant, rendering the medication less effective—or entirely ineffective—against future infections. This means that individuals who rely on antibiotics repeatedly to treat UTIs may find themselves facing a situation where their infections become more difficult to treat, leading to a vicious cycle of recurring infections and escalating antibiotic use.

The Growing Problem of Antibiotic Resistance

Antibiotic resistance is not just an abstract concept; it's a real and escalating issue. In fact, the Centers for Disease Control and Prevention (CDC) reports that antibiotic-resistant infections are responsible for at least 2.8 million infections and 35,000 deaths annually in the U.S. alone. The problem is exacerbated by the overprescription of antibiotics for conditions that may not even require them, such as viral infections or mild bacterial infections that could resolve on their own. When antibiotics are used unnecessarily, they contribute to the development of resistant bacteria, putting individuals at greater risk of serious infections in the future.

Additionally, the misuse of antibiotics, such as stopping treatment too early or not following the prescribed dosage, can lead to partial bacterial eradication, allowing resistant bacteria to survive and thrive.

Rethinking Antibiotic Use

While antibiotics are a necessary tool in treating many infections, including UTIs, their overuse has led us to rethink how and when they should be used. For individuals prone to recurrent UTIs, it's essential to adopt a more mindful approach to antibiotic use—one that prioritizes their effectiveness while minimizing the risks associated with overuse.

When Antibiotics Are Necessary

Antibiotics are essential for treating active UTIs caused by bacterial infections, and they should be used appropriately under the guidance of a healthcare provider. If you are experiencing symptoms such as painful urination, frequent urges to urinate, lower abdominal pain, or blood in your urine, it's important to seek medical attention and get a proper diagnosis. A healthcare provider can determine if an antibiotic is necessary and recommend the most appropriate treatment for the specific bacteria causing the infection.

However, antibiotics should not be relied upon as a first-line solution for every UTI. For individuals who experience recurrent infections, it's crucial to explore other treatment options alongside antibiotics to prevent the need for repeated courses. Overusing antibiotics can lead to complications, including antibiotic resistance, yeast infections, and a disrupted gut microbiome.

Using Antibiotics Wisely

When antibiotics are necessary, it's essential to use them responsibly. Always follow your healthcare provider's instructions regarding dosage, timing, and the duration of treatment. Do not stop taking antibiotics prematurely, even if your symptoms improve, as doing so can result in incomplete bacterial eradication and contribute to resistance.

Moreover, it's essential to avoid taking antibiotics for conditions where they won't help. Antibiotics are ineffective against viral infections like colds or the flu, and unnecessary use in these cases can contribute to the growing resistance problem.

Incorporating a more holistic approach to managing UTIs—one that includes lifestyle changes, preventive strategies, and complementary treatments—can reduce the frequency and severity of infections, minimizing the need for antibiotics.

Strategies for Managing Antibiotic Resistance

Managing antibiotic resistance involves taking proactive steps to avoid the cycle of recurring UTIs and reduce reliance on antibiotics. By adopting a comprehensive approach that focuses on prevention, lifestyle changes, and natural remedies, you can reduce your chances of developing infections and limit the need for antibiotics.

Prevention Is Key

As the saying goes, "An ounce of prevention is worth a pound of cure." By focusing on prevention, you can reduce the frequency of UTIs and minimize your reliance on antibiotics. The strategies discussed in previous chapters—such as staying hydrated, practicing good hygiene, eating a bladder-friendly diet, and incorporating probiotics into your routine—

are all essential components of a prevention-focused approach.

By taking these preventative steps, you can support your urinary system, strengthen your immune defenses, and reduce the risk of infection. The less frequently you experience UTIs, the less often you'll need antibiotics.

Probiotics and Natural Supplements
Probiotics and natural supplements play an important role in supporting bladder health and preventing infections. Probiotic-rich foods like yogurt, kefir, and fermented vegetables help promote a healthy balance of bacteria in your urinary tract, preventing harmful bacteria from proliferating. Certain natural supplements, such as cranberry extract, D-mannose, and uva ursi, may also provide support in preventing UTIs by making the urinary tract less hospitable to harmful bacteria.

Incorporating these natural strategies into your routine may not only reduce your need for antibiotics but also provide ongoing support for your urinary system, helping you maintain long-term health.

Mind-Body Techniques for Stress Management

Stress can weaken your immune system and make you more susceptible to infections. Incorporating mind-body techniques like meditation, deep breathing exercises, and yoga can help you manage stress, improve emotional well-being, and enhance overall health. These practices can help reduce the impact of stress on your body, making it easier to manage the physical and emotional burden of recurrent UTIs.

Additionally, stress reduction practices can help address the underlying emotional factors that may contribute to the cycle of recurring infections. By fostering emotional resilience, you can support your physical healing process and reduce your dependence on antibiotics.

Conclusion: Finding a Balanced Approach

Antibiotics play a crucial role in treating UTIs, but they are not a long-term solution for recurrent infections. Overuse of antibiotics has led to the growing problem of antibiotic resistance, which poses a serious threat to public health. By adopting a more mindful approach to antibiotic use—focusing on prevention, natural remedies, and lifestyle changes—you can reduce your reliance on antibiotics and break the cycle of recurring infections.

Chapter 5

Practical Tools to Track and Tackle Your UTI Journey

One of the most effective ways to take control of your health and reduce the recurrence of urinary tract infections (UTIs) is through tracking and understanding your body's patterns. By documenting symptoms, triggers, and lifestyle habits, you can pinpoint the root causes of recurrent infections and take targeted actions toward healing. In this chapter, we will explore practical tools that can help you track your UTI journey, including a symptom tracker, a daily healing journal, and goal-setting strategies to guide you toward a UTI-free life.

Creating Your Symptom Tracker

A symptom tracker is an invaluable tool for anyone dealing with recurrent UTIs. By documenting your symptoms over time, you can begin to identify patterns and potential triggers that might be contributing to your infections. Understanding these patterns is key to preventing future flare-ups and reducing reliance on antibiotics.

How to Track Your Symptoms Effectively
When creating your symptom tracker, it's important to record several key factors. This can include:

1. **Date and Time**: Track when you first notice symptoms, how long they last, and any fluctuations you experience throughout the day.

2. **Symptom Type**: Document the exact symptoms you experience, such as pain or burning during urination, frequent urges to urinate, blood in the urine, lower abdominal pain, cloudy or foul-smelling urine, and fatigue.

3. **Severity**: Rate the severity of each symptom on a scale from 1-10. This can help you notice shifts in the intensity of

your symptoms, providing insight into how your body is responding to different lifestyle changes or treatments.

4. **Triggers**: Note any potential triggers that might contribute to your symptoms. This can include dietary factors, stressful events, new medications, hygiene habits, or exposure to environmental irritants.

5. **Treatment or Remedies**: Record any treatments you try, including over-the-counter medications, antibiotics, natural remedies (like cranberry supplements or probiotics), and any lifestyle changes (like increased hydration or dietary modifications). Track whether these treatments seem to alleviate or worsen your symptoms.

Why Tracking Matters

By consistently tracking your symptoms, you can identify recurring patterns that may point to underlying causes—whether it's a particular food, a period of heightened stress, or a certain hygiene practice. Tracking your symptoms over time can also help you determine the effectiveness of various treatments, giving you valuable insights into what works best for your body.

Daily Healing Journal

Your healing journey isn't just about physical symptoms—it's also about emotional and mental well-being. Chronic UTIs can take a toll on your emotional health, contributing to stress, frustration, and feelings of isolation. That's why it's important to maintain a **Daily Healing Journal** that goes beyond tracking physical symptoms and incorporates your emotional, mental, and social health.

Guided Exercises for Holistic Healing

Your Daily Healing Journal can include guided exercises designed to promote emotional healing, enhance self-awareness, and keep you focused on your health goals. Here are some prompts you can include in your journal:

1. **Hydration Log**: Track your daily water intake to ensure you're staying adequately hydrated. This is a simple yet

effective way to support your bladder health and help prevent infections.

2. **Diet and Nutrition Tracking**: Keep a log of the foods you eat each day, and note any foods that may trigger your symptoms. Pay attention to foods that promote bladder health (like cranberries, probiotics, and fiber) and avoid those that can irritate the bladder (such as caffeine, spicy foods, or artificial sweeteners).

3. **Emotional Check-In**: Begin or end each day by noting how you feel emotionally. Are you feeling stressed, anxious, or overwhelmed? Emotional health plays a critical role in overall well-being, so acknowledging your feelings can help you manage stress and anxiety, which may contribute to recurring infections.

4. **Physical Symptoms**: Document how your physical symptoms are progressing. Are they improving with certain changes in diet or lifestyle? Are you experiencing any flare-ups? This section can help you

correlate your symptoms with the lifestyle choices you're making.

5. **Mind-Body Practices**: Reflect on any relaxation or stress-relief techniques you incorporate into your daily routine, such as meditation, yoga, deep breathing, or journaling. These practices can help lower stress levels and support your immune system, which is crucial for preventing infections.

The Power of Consistency

The key to a successful healing journal is consistency. Try to write in your journal every day—ideally at the same time each day—so that you can track your progress, identify patterns, and stay mindful of the emotional and physical aspects of your healing journey. Journaling is a powerful tool for emotional release, self-reflection, and personal growth, all of which contribute to long-term health.

Setting Healing Goals

Setting clear, actionable goals is essential for anyone looking to break free from the cycle of recurrent UTIs. By identifying specific, measurable goals and taking small, consistent steps toward them, you can empower yourself and create lasting change. Healing is a journey, and setting goals will help you stay focused and motivated along the way.

Actionable Steps for a UTI-Free Life

Here are some steps you can take every day to reduce your risk of future infections:

1. **Hydration Goal**: Aim to drink at least 8 glasses of water per day. Proper hydration flushes out bacteria from the urinary tract and helps maintain bladder health. Consider setting a daily reminder on your phone to help you stay on track.

2. **Dietary Goal**: Make it a goal to include more bladder-friendly foods in your diet. This might mean incorporating more probiotics, fiber-rich foods, and antioxidants into your meals, while avoiding foods that trigger irritation, like caffeine or spicy foods.

3. **Mind-Body Practices**: Set a goal to engage in a stress-reducing activity for at least 10-15 minutes each day. Whether it's meditation, yoga, or simply deep breathing, these practices can help calm your mind and reduce the emotional strain that can contribute to UTIs.

4. **Physical Activity**: Exercise can help promote healthy circulation and support your immune system. Set a realistic goal for physical activity, whether it's a daily walk, yoga session, or more intense workouts, to keep your body strong and resilient.

5. **Regular UTI Check-Ins**: Set a goal to check in with your healthcare provider or a specialist if your symptoms persist or worsen. Tracking your symptoms and sharing the information with your healthcare provider can help you make informed decisions about treatment and lifestyle changes.

Small Steps, Big Results
When setting healing goals, make sure they are

specific, achievable, and aligned with your long-term health aspirations. Breaking down your larger goal of living a UTI-free life into small, manageable steps will help you stay motivated and on track. These goals should be revisited regularly to assess progress and make adjustments as needed.

Conclusion: Empowering Your Healing Journey

Tracking your symptoms, journaling your experiences, and setting clear, actionable goals are essential tools for tackling recurrent UTIs. By combining these practical tools with the holistic approaches outlined in this book, you can take control of your health and work toward a life free from frequent infections. Remember, healing is not just about eliminating physical symptoms—it's about nurturing your emotional well-being and making empowered choices every day.

Chapter 6

The Emotional Impact: Healing Beyond the Physical Symptoms

While dealing with recurrent urinary tract infections (UTIs) often focuses on the physical symptoms, the emotional toll of living with this condition can be just as significant. The frustration of frequent infections, the isolation caused by ongoing health struggles, and the fear of never finding a solution can deeply affect your mental and emotional well-being. This chapter will explore the emotional impact of living with recurrent UTIs, offer practical exercises to help build emotional resilience and self-compassion, and emphasize the importance of connecting with others who understand your journey.

Addressing the Emotional Toll

The mental health challenges that come with recurrent UTIs are often overlooked, but they are just as important as the physical symptoms. Chronic UTIs can trigger a range of emotions, including frustration, isolation, fear, and hopelessness. These emotional struggles can compound the physical pain and contribute to an overwhelming sense of being stuck in an endless cycle of infections and treatments.

The Emotional Strain of Recurring Infections

Living with recurrent UTIs often feels like a constant battle. The unpredictability of symptoms, the constant fear of another infection, and the perceived lack of effective treatments can leave you feeling helpless and exhausted. Many people with chronic conditions, such as UTIs, experience feelings of frustration when treatments don't seem to work or when they are met with medical dismissal. This can lead to a sense of hopelessness and emotional exhaustion.

The fear of never fully healing, especially when infections keep recurring, can create a deep sense of anxiety. There's also the emotional toll of social isolation—avoiding social events due to symptoms or not feeling comfortable talking about your condition with others. These feelings of isolation can leave you feeling misunderstood and disconnected from your support network.

Coping with Frustration and Anxiety

It's important to recognize that your emotional response to recurrent UTIs is valid. Feeling frustrated and anxious is a natural reaction to chronic illness. However, it's essential to develop healthy coping mechanisms to manage these emotions. Strategies such as mindfulness, stress-relief techniques, and emotional support can be incredibly beneficial in reducing anxiety and helping you regain a sense of control.

Building Resilience

Building emotional resilience doesn't mean ignoring your struggles; it means acknowledging them and developing coping strategies that allow you to face the challenges of living with recurrent UTIs. Emotional resilience is the ability to bounce back from adversity, adapt to change, and maintain a sense of inner strength during difficult times. Here are some practical exercises to help you build resilience throughout your healing journey:

1. Mindfulness and Meditation
Mindfulness practices can help you stay present and focused, rather than becoming overwhelmed by the future or past. Practicing mindfulness allows you to accept your emotions without judgment and reduces anxiety by grounding you in the present moment.

- **Exercise**: Set aside 10-15 minutes each day to practice mindfulness meditation. Focus on your breath, gently guiding your thoughts back to your breath if your mind wanders. This practice can help reduce stress, lower anxiety, and create a sense of calm.

2. Breathing Exercises for Stress Relief
When you feel overwhelmed, deep breathing

exercises can be an immediate way to calm your body and mind. By slowing down your breathing, you activate the parasympathetic nervous system, which counteracts the fight-or-flight response, helping to alleviate stress.

- **Exercise**: Practice diaphragmatic breathing, also known as deep belly breathing. Breathe in deeply through your nose for a count of four, hold for four counts, and then exhale slowly through your mouth for a count of six. Repeat this for several minutes to release tension.

3. Journaling for Emotional Clarity

Journaling is a powerful tool for emotional processing. Writing down your thoughts and feelings allows you to gain clarity, release pent-up emotions, and develop a deeper understanding of your mental and emotional state. Journaling can also be an effective way to track your progress and celebrate your small victories.

- **Exercise**: Each day, write down your emotions. You might ask yourself questions like, "How am I feeling today?",

"What is causing me stress?", or "What am I grateful for today?" Reflect on your answers to help process your emotions and identify areas where you can build resilience.

4. Self-Compassion Practices

Self-compassion is about being kind and understanding toward yourself, especially during times of struggle. Many people with chronic conditions tend to be their harshest critics, but cultivating self-compassion can reduce feelings of guilt and shame and improve emotional well-being.

- **Exercise**: Practice speaking kindly to yourself as you would to a friend. When you feel frustrated or defeated, remind yourself that it's okay to have tough days. Offer yourself comfort and reassurance, acknowledging that healing is a journey, not a destination.

5. Celebrating Small Wins

Building resilience also involves recognizing and celebrating your progress, no matter how small. Every step forward—whether it's managing a flare-up more effectively, reducing stress, or making healthier lifestyle choices—is an achievement. Acknowledging these moments fosters a sense of accomplishment and motivation to continue the journey.

- **Exercise**: Keep a "Small Wins" journal. Each time you experience a victory, big or small, write it down. Reflect on how far you've come, and take pride in your ability to adapt and persevere.

Connecting with Others

One of the most powerful ways to heal emotionally is to connect with others who understand what you're going through. Chronic conditions like recurrent UTIs can feel isolating, especially if friends and family don't fully grasp the emotional toll of the condition. Finding or creating support networks can help you feel seen, heard, and less alone in your journey.

The Importance of Community
Being part of a community where others share similar experiences can provide immense

emotional support. These communities offer a safe space to express your fears, frustrations, and triumphs. Sharing your journey with others who understand can help reduce feelings of isolation, encourage empathy, and provide practical tips and emotional support.

Where to Find Support

There are numerous resources and communities available for individuals dealing with recurrent UTIs. These may include:

1. **Online Support Groups**: Websites like Facebook, Reddit, and dedicated health forums have private support groups where individuals can share experiences, advice, and emotional support.

2. **Local Support Groups**: Many hospitals, clinics, or nonprofit organizations offer in-person support groups for individuals dealing with chronic conditions. These can provide an opportunity for face-to-face support and a sense of camaraderie.

3. **Healthcare Providers**: Some doctors or therapists specialize in emotional health for people with chronic illnesses. Seeking professional guidance can help you address feelings of depression, anxiety, or frustration that arise from living with recurrent UTIs.

Creating Your Own Community

If you can't find a support group that fits your needs, consider creating your own. This could be a virtual group, a local meetup, or even a small group of friends or family members who understand your journey and offer support.

The Power of Shared Experiences

Hearing from others who have navigated the same challenges can be incredibly empowering. Real-life stories from those who have successfully managed their condition, made lifestyle changes, or found alternative treatments can inspire hope and help you see that you are not alone.

Conclusion: Healing Beyond the Physical

While managing recurrent UTIs requires attention to physical health, it's equally important to address the emotional impact of the condition. Building emotional resilience, practicing self-compassion, and connecting with others can transform your healing journey from one of isolation and frustration to one of empowerment and community. By integrating these emotional support strategies, you can not only heal your body but also nurture your emotional well-being, ultimately leading to a healthier, more balanced life.

Chapter 7

Understanding Your Body: The Science Behind UTIs

Urinary tract infections (UTIs) are common yet often misunderstood. To truly take control of your healing journey, it's crucial to understand what's happening inside your body when you experience a UTI, why some people are more susceptible to recurrent infections, and how UTIs can affect more than just your bladder. In this chapter, we'll break down the science of UTIs in simple terms, explore the anatomy of these infections, and look at the broader implications they can have on your overall health.

What's Happening When You Have a UTI?

A urinary tract infection (UTI) occurs when harmful bacteria enter the urinary tract and begin to multiply. This can lead to inflammation, irritation, and symptoms like burning during urination, frequent urges to go, and cloudy or foul-smelling urine. The urinary tract is made up of several parts, including the kidneys, bladder, ureters, and urethra, and any part of this system can become infected. Most UTIs affect the lower urinary tract—specifically the bladder and urethra.

The infection typically begins when bacteria, often from the skin or rectal area, travel into the urethra and move up into the bladder. The body's immune system then tries to fight off the bacteria, which causes the inflammation and discomfort you feel. In some cases, the infection can spread further up into the kidneys, which can lead to more severe symptoms and complications, such as pyelonephritis (kidney infection).

Understanding the basic process of infection helps you appreciate why prevention and early treatment are so important. Untreated UTIs can lead to serious complications, including kidney damage or sepsis, a life-threatening condition where the body's response to infection becomes widespread.

The Anatomy of a UTI

To understand why UTIs happen, it's essential to know how the urinary system works and why some individuals are more prone to recurrent infections.

1. The Urinary Tract:
The urinary tract consists of several parts:

- **Kidneys**: Filter waste and excess fluid from the blood.

- **Ureters**: Tubes that carry urine from the kidneys to the bladder.

- **Bladder**: A storage sac that holds urine until it's eliminated from the body.

- **Urethra**: A tube that carries urine from the bladder to the outside of the body.

2. How Infections Occur:
The most common cause of UTIs is the introduction of bacteria into the urethra, usually from the skin or bowel. From there, the bacteria can ascend into the bladder. The body's natural

defenses, such as urination, help to flush out bacteria, but in some cases, the bacteria can evade these defenses and multiply, leading to infection.

Why Are Some People More Susceptible?

Several factors can increase the likelihood of developing recurrent UTIs, including:

- **Anatomical Differences**: Women have a shorter urethra than men, which makes it easier for bacteria to travel into the bladder.

- **Urinary Retention**: Not emptying the bladder completely can allow bacteria to grow and cause infection.

- **Hormonal Changes**: Hormonal fluctuations, such as those during pregnancy or menopause, can affect urinary tract health.

- **Chronic Medical Conditions**: Conditions like diabetes or a weakened immune system can make it harder for the body to fight off infections.

- **Sexual Activity**: Sexual intercourse can introduce bacteria into the urinary tract.

- **Urinary Catheters**: Catheters increase the risk of UTIs due to the introduction of bacteria into the urinary tract.

While UTIs are common in the general population, some individuals are more prone to developing them repeatedly. If you've experienced recurrent UTIs, understanding these risk factors can help guide you toward better prevention strategies and more effective treatments.

How UTIs Can Affect More Than Your Bladder

Most people associate UTIs with bladder discomfort, but untreated or recurrent infections can lead to more serious complications that affect your entire body. It's important to recognize that a UTI is not just a localized issue—if left untreated, it can spread and impact other areas of your health.

1. Kidney Infections (Pyelonephritis):

If a UTI is not treated, it can spread up the ureters into the kidneys, leading to pyelonephritis. This can cause severe symptoms, including high fever, chills, nausea, vomiting, and back pain. Kidney infections can lead to permanent kidney damage if not addressed promptly.

2. Sepsis:

In rare cases, untreated UTIs can lead to sepsis, a life-threatening condition where the infection spreads throughout the body and triggers widespread inflammation. Sepsis can cause organ failure and, if not treated immediately, can be fatal.

3. Impact on the Immune System:

Frequent or chronic UTIs can take a toll on your immune system. The constant battle between your body's immune cells and the bacteria can weaken your immune defenses, making it harder for your body to fight off other infections. Chronic inflammation caused by recurring UTIs can also contribute to overall fatigue, and long-term immune system strain.

4. Emotional and Mental Health:

The physical pain and discomfort caused by recurrent UTIs can lead to significant emotional and mental strain. The stress of managing chronic infections, the anxiety of frequent flare-ups, and the fear of recurrence can take a toll on your emotional health. Depression, anxiety, and frustration are common emotional side effects of dealing with a long-term illness like recurrent UTIs.

5. Sexual Health:

Frequent UTIs can also affect your sexual health. Many people with recurrent UTIs find that sexual activity triggers infections, and the fear of developing a UTI after intercourse can lead to avoidance of intimacy. This, in turn, can cause relationship strain and feelings of frustration or isolation.

6. Bladder Health:

Chronic UTIs can lead to bladder changes, including bladder overactivity or a condition known as interstitial cystitis. This condition causes persistent bladder pain, urgency, and frequency, and can become a long-term issue if recurrent UTIs are not properly managed.

The Importance of a Multi-Faceted Approach to Healing

Understanding the broader impact of recurrent UTIs emphasizes the need for a comprehensive, multi-faceted approach to healing. It's not just about treating the infection at hand—it's about addressing the root causes, managing the symptoms, and preventing future infections.

While antibiotics are often necessary to clear up acute infections, relying solely on them may not address the underlying reasons for recurrent UTIs. It's important to adopt a holistic approach that includes:

- **Lifestyle Modifications**: Incorporating hydration, healthy diet, and hygiene practices into your daily routine.

- **Mind-Body Techniques**: Stress management through techniques like meditation, yoga, and breathing exercises to reduce the emotional toll of chronic illness.

- **Nutrition**: Certain foods and supplements can support urinary tract health and prevent infections.

- **Emotional Healing**: Addressing the emotional impact of living with recurrent UTIs through journaling, therapy, and connecting with support networks.

A comprehensive approach, which combines both medical treatments and holistic self-care strategies, will give you the tools needed to manage and prevent future UTIs more effectively. Understanding the science behind UTIs empowers you to take an active role in your health, make informed decisions, and feel more in control of your journey toward healing.

Conclusion

By understanding the science behind UTIs, you're better equipped to recognize how these infections affect more than just your bladder. You've learned about the anatomy of a UTI, why some people are more susceptible, and the broader impact untreated or recurrent infections can have on your body. With this knowledge, you can begin to approach your healing journey with a clearer sense of purpose and direction, knowing that prevention, holistic care, and self-awareness are key to long-term success.

Chapter 8

Exploring Natural Remedies: What Really Works?

For anyone who has suffered from recurrent UTIs, the frustration is palpable. You do everything right—stay hydrated, practice good hygiene, even take antibiotics—but the infections keep coming back. This cycle of pain, burning, and disruption to daily life can feel endless.

Naturally, many people turn to alternative and natural remedies in the hope of breaking free from this relentless pattern. The internet is flooded with suggestions, from cranberry juice to herbal teas, but how do you separate fact from fiction? More importantly, can natural remedies truly provide lasting relief, or are they just another temporary fix? In this chapter, we'll dive deep into the world of natural solutions— what works, what doesn't, and how to use these remedies wisely as part of a holistic strategy for healing and prevention.

Herbal Solutions and Supplements

Nature has long provided us with powerful tools for healing, and when it comes to bladder and urinary tract health, certain herbs and supplements have shown promise. Below, we explore some of the most researched and effective options:

1. D-Mannose: The UTI Game Changer

D-Mannose, a type of sugar found in fruits like cranberries, has gained attention for its ability to prevent bacteria (especially *E. coli*) from sticking to the bladder wall. Clinical studies suggest that taking D-Mannose regularly may help reduce the recurrence of UTIs, making it a go-to option for those seeking a natural preventative approach.

2. Cranberry Extract: Beyond the Juice

While cranberry juice has been widely touted as a UTI remedy, its high sugar content can sometimes do more harm than good. However, cranberry extract supplements contain concentrated levels of proanthocyanidins (PACs), which may help prevent bacterial adhesion in the bladder. It's important to choose a high-quality extract with a standardized amount of PACs to ensure effectiveness.

3. Uva Ursi (Bearberry Leaf): A Natural Antiseptic

Uva Ursi has been used in traditional medicine for its antibacterial properties. Its active compound, arbutin, breaks down into hydroquinone, which has antimicrobial effects. However, Uva Ursi should be used with caution, as long-term use may be harmful to the liver.

4. Garlic Extract: A Potent Antimicrobial

Garlic contains allicin, a natural compound with strong antibacterial properties. Some studies suggest that garlic extract may help combat antibiotic-resistant bacteria, making it a potential complementary remedy for those struggling with recurrent infections.

5. Probiotics: Restoring Balance

A healthy urinary tract depends on a balanced microbiome. Probiotics, particularly *Lactobacillus* strains, can help maintain healthy vaginal and bladder flora, reducing the risk of harmful bacterial overgrowth. Taking probiotics regularly may support overall urinary tract health and enhance the body's natural defenses against infection.

Home Remedies That Work

Many home remedies are passed down through generations, but do they truly help with UTIs? Let's explore some natural at-home strategies that can provide real relief:

1. Hydration: The Most Overlooked Solution

Drinking plenty of water helps flush bacteria from the bladder before they have a chance to multiply. Aiming for at least 8-10 glasses of water per day can make a significant difference in both prevention and symptom relief.

2. Baking Soda: Fact or Fiction?

Some people swear by baking soda as a way to neutralize urine acidity and relieve burning sensations. While this may provide temporary relief, excessive use of baking soda can disrupt the body's pH balance and lead to unwanted side effects.

3. Apple Cider Vinegar: A Double-Edged Sword

Apple cider vinegar has antibacterial properties, but drinking it in excess can irritate the bladder. If used, it should be heavily diluted and consumed in moderation.

4. Heat Therapy: Soothing Pain Naturally

A warm compress on the lower abdomen can provide immediate relief from UTI-related discomfort by relaxing muscles and reducing cramping.

5. Avoiding Bladder Irritants

Caffeine, alcohol, and acidic foods can worsen symptoms. Reducing or eliminating these irritants from your diet during an active infection can support healing and prevent further irritation.

Understanding the Limits of Natural Remedies

While natural remedies can be incredibly helpful in supporting urinary tract health, it is crucial to understand their limitations. Here's why:

1. They Don't Work for Severe Infections

If a UTI has already progressed into a kidney infection, natural remedies alone are not sufficient. Signs such as fever, chills, back pain, and nausea indicate that medical intervention is necessary.

2. They Should Complement, Not Replace, Medical Treatment

While natural solutions can help prevent and manage mild UTIs, they should not be used as a sole treatment for ongoing or severe infections. Antibiotics remain the most effective way to treat acute bacterial infections.

3. Not All Natural Remedies Are Safe for Everyone

Herbal remedies can interact with medications and may not be suitable for people with certain medical conditions. Consulting a healthcare professional before starting any new supplement or natural treatment is always recommended.

4. Consistency is Key

Many natural remedies require regular, long-term use before results are noticeable. Unlike antibiotics, which act quickly, natural approaches often work more slowly and require patience.

A Balanced Approach to Healing

The key to successfully managing UTIs is a balanced approach—integrating natural remedies with medical care, lifestyle changes, and self-care strategies.

Chapter 9

Long-Term UTI Management – Sustainable Strategies for a UTI-Free Life

Living with the fear of recurring urinary tract infections (UTIs) can feel like walking on a tightrope—constantly worrying about the next infection, second-guessing your habits, and wondering if there's a way to break free from the cycle. The good news? You don't have to live in fear forever. Managing UTIs isn't just about treating them when they happen—it's about building a lifestyle that prevents them from coming back. In this chapter, we'll explore sustainable, long-term strategies to help you reclaim your health, feel confident in your body, and enjoy life without the looming shadow of another UTI.

Building Sustainable Habits

The key to long-term UTI prevention is consistency. Small, daily actions—when done consistently—create a strong defense against recurring infections. Unlike temporary solutions, sustainable habits work to strengthen your body's natural ability to fight off bacteria before they cause an infection.

1. Hydration as a Daily Practice

Drinking enough water is one of the simplest, yet most powerful, ways to prevent UTIs. Hydration helps flush out bacteria before they have a chance to settle and multiply in the urinary tract.

Action Step:

- Carry a reusable water bottle and aim for at least 8-10 glasses of water daily.

- Set reminders on your phone to drink water throughout the day.

- Infuse your water with lemon or cucumber if plain water feels boring.

2. Prioritizing Bladder Health with Nutrition

What you eat has a direct impact on your urinary tract health. A diet rich in bladder-friendly foods can support the immune system, reduce inflammation, and create an environment where harmful bacteria struggle to thrive.

Foods That Support Bladder Health:
✓ Cranberries (contain compounds that prevent bacteria from sticking to the bladder wall)
✓ Probiotic-rich foods (like yogurt, kefir, sauerkraut) to support gut and urinary health
✓ Leafy greens (reduce inflammation and provide essential vitamins)
✓ Garlic and turmeric (natural antimicrobial properties)
✓ Berries (packed with antioxidants to support the immune system)

Foods to Minimize or Avoid:
✗ Excessive caffeine (can irritate the bladder)
✗ Sugary drinks and processed foods (can fuel bacterial overgrowth)
✗ Alcohol (can dehydrate and irritate the urinary tract)

Action Step:

- Keep a food journal to identify any triggers that might worsen bladder symptoms.

- Incorporate at least one bladder-supportive food into your diet each day.

- Experiment with herbal teas like marshmallow root or dandelion for bladder soothing.

3. Maintaining Healthy Bathroom Habits

It might seem simple, but your bathroom habits play a significant role in UTI prevention.

✓ Urinate regularly (don't hold it in for long periods).
✓ Wipe front to back to prevent bacteria from entering the urethra.
✓ Empty your bladder after sexual activity to flush out bacteria.
✓ Avoid harsh soaps or douches in the genital area to maintain a healthy pH balance.

Action Step:

- Pay attention to your body's signals and make urination a priority.

- Create a gentle hygiene routine using mild, fragrance-free products.

The Power of Consistency

Many people adopt good habits after experiencing a UTI, only to slip back into old patterns once they feel better. This cycle often leads to another infection. The true key to a UTI-free life is making these habits a permanent part of your daily routine.

1. Tracking Your Health Over Time

Keeping a health journal or symptom tracker can help identify patterns and potential triggers for your UTIs.

Action Step:

- Record your daily water intake, diet, bathroom habits, and any symptoms in a journal.

- Note any stressful events, travel, or dietary changes that coincide with infections.

- Use this information to adjust your habits and take proactive steps before an infection occurs.

2. Regular Medical Checkups

Even if you're following all the right steps, it's still important to check in with your healthcare provider regularly—especially if you've had multiple UTIs in the past year.

Action Step:

- Schedule routine urine tests to catch any bacterial growth early.

- Discuss long-term prevention strategies with your doctor, such as low-dose antibiotics (if necessary) or alternative therapies.

- If UTIs are persistent, request a referral to a urologist for further evaluation.

Living with Confidence

One of the most challenging aspects of recurrent UTIs is the mental toll they take. Many people live in fear—canceling plans, avoiding intimacy, or feeling anxious about every minor twinge in their bladder. This fear can be just as debilitating as the infections themselves.

1. Letting Go of Anxiety Around UTIs

Chronic UTIs often lead to health anxiety, where every sensation in the bladder feels like the start of another infection. Learning to manage this anxiety can help you feel in control of your body again.

Mind-Body Techniques to Reduce Anxiety:
Deep Breathing: Practicing diaphragmatic breathing can calm the nervous system and prevent stress-induced bladder irritation.
Guided Meditation: Listening to a relaxation meditation can help rewire your brain's fear response.
Journaling: Writing about your fears and frustrations can help release the emotional weight of chronic infections.

Action Step:

- Try a 5-minute deep breathing exercise when you feel anxious about your bladder.

- Write down three things you're grateful for in your health each morning.

2. Rebuilding Trust in Your Body

After repeated infections, it's easy to feel like your body is working against you. However, by consistently caring for your urinary tract health, you can rebuild that trust and start feeling confident again.

Action Step:

- Celebrate small victories, like a month without a UTI.

- Shift your focus from "fear of infections" to "appreciation for wellness."

- Surround yourself with a supportive community that understands your journey.

Final Thoughts: Taking Ownership of Your Health

Long-term UTI management isn't about one magic solution—it's about adopting a lifestyle that makes infections less likely to return. The power lies in your hands. With the right habits, awareness, and mindset, you can break free from the cycle of recurrent UTIs and step into a future where your health isn't defined by infections but by confidence, resilience, and lasting well-being.

Chapter 10

The Common Solutions You've Tried— And Why They Don't Work

If you're reading this chapter, chances are you've already tried multiple solutions to get rid of your UTIs—and yet, they keep coming back. The cycle of infection, treatment, and recurrence is exhausting, frustrating, and sometimes downright demoralizing. It's not just about the physical symptoms; it's the emotional toll of constantly worrying about the next infection, feeling dismissed by doctors, and wondering if you'll ever find a real solution.

Many of the most common treatments seem logical on the surface but fail to address the root causes of chronic UTIs. Some provide only temporary relief, while others may even contribute to long-term harm, like antibiotic resistance or imbalances in the body. Let's break down the most commonly tried solutions, why they don't work in the long run, and what you can do instead.

Antibiotics: A Double-Edged Sword

For decades, antibiotics have been the go-to treatment for UTIs. While they can effectively kill off the bacteria causing an active infection, they don't address why the infection occurred in the first place. This is why so many people end up in a frustrating cycle of recurring infections.

Here's why antibiotics aren't a long-term fix:

- **They don't prevent future infections.** Once the course of antibiotics ends, bacteria can easily return—especially if the underlying issues (like imbalanced vaginal microbiome or bladder inflammation) aren't addressed.

- **They kill beneficial bacteria.** Antibiotics don't just target harmful bacteria; they also wipe out the good bacteria that help maintain a balanced urinary and vaginal microbiome. This can leave you more vulnerable to future infections.

- **Antibiotic resistance is real.** Repeated use of antibiotics can lead to resistant bacteria, making future infections harder to treat. This means stronger medications, longer recovery times, and more potential side effects.

So, while antibiotics can be necessary for severe infections, relying on them as the primary strategy for UTI management is not a sustainable solution.

Cranberry Supplements or Juice: Not the Magic Cure

Cranberries have been hyped as a natural UTI remedy for years, but research on their effectiveness is mixed. While some studies suggest that cranberry compounds (proanthocyanidins) may prevent certain bacteria from sticking to the bladder lining, they don't kill bacteria or treat an active infection.

Why cranberries fall short:

- **Most cranberry products are too weak.** Many commercial juices contain added sugar, which can actually worsen UTIs, and supplements often lack enough of the active ingredient to be effective.

- **They don't work once an infection has started.** Even if cranberry helps prevent bacteria from sticking, it won't clear an infection that has already taken hold.

- **Not everyone benefits from them.** The effectiveness of cranberry varies by person, and many find no relief at all.

Over-the-Counter Urinary Pain Relief Medications (e.g., Pyridium, Azo)

Medications like phenazopyridine (Pyridium, Azo) can be a lifesaver when you're dealing with UTI pain, burning, and urgency. But here's the problem—they don't treat the infection.

Why these meds aren't enough:

- **They only mask symptoms.** You might feel better for a few hours, but the bacteria are still present and multiplying.

- **They don't address the root cause.** While symptom relief is important, these meds won't stop recurrent infections from happening.

- **They can give a false sense of security.** Feeling better might delay seeking proper treatment, allowing the infection to worsen.

Home Remedies (e.g., Drinking More Water, Using Heat Pads)

Many people try simple home remedies to manage UTIs, and while some may help with comfort, they aren't real solutions.

- **Drinking more water helps flush bacteria, but it's not enough to kill an infection.** Hydration is important, but water alone won't eliminate a bacterial infection that has already taken hold.

- **Heat pads may soothe pain, but they don't treat the underlying problem.** They can provide temporary relief from bladder discomfort, but they don't kill bacteria or prevent recurrence.

Probiotics: Helpful but Not a Standalone Solution

Probiotics are often recommended to restore good bacteria in the gut and vaginal microbiome, which can play a role in UTI prevention. However, they aren't a guaranteed fix.

- **Not all probiotics target the urinary tract.** Many generic probiotics focus on gut health, which won't necessarily benefit bladder health.

- **They need to be used consistently.** Probiotics don't work overnight, and their effects depend on your overall diet and lifestyle.

- **They don't treat active infections.** While they may help with prevention, probiotics won't clear an existing infection.

Frequent Bathroom Visits to "Flush" the Infection

Many people believe that urinating frequently will help flush out bacteria and stop a UTI. While staying hydrated is important, frequent urination won't eliminate bacteria that have already attached to the bladder wall.

- **Bacteria can cling to bladder cells.** Once an infection starts, urinating more won't be enough to remove the bacteria.

- **It can worsen irritation.** Constantly trying to urinate when the bladder is inflamed can make symptoms feel worse.

Antibiotic Prophylaxis (Long-Term Low-Dose Antibiotics)

Some doctors prescribe low-dose antibiotics as a preventive measure, but this approach is problematic.

- **It leads to antibiotic resistance.** Long-term antibiotic use can make bacteria more resistant, making future infections harder to treat.

- **It disrupts the microbiome.** Chronic antibiotic use can throw off the balance of bacteria in the body, leading to yeast infections and gut issues.

- **It's not sustainable.** Relying on daily antibiotics forever is not a healthy or effective long-term strategy.

D-Mannose Supplements: Limited Effectiveness

D-Mannose is a sugar that can prevent certain bacteria (like E. coli) from sticking to the bladder wall. Some people find it helpful, but it's not a universal cure.

- **It doesn't work for all types of UTIs.** Not all UTIs are caused by E. coli, and D-Mannose is ineffective against other bacteria.

- **It won't treat an active infection.** Like cranberries, it may help prevent infection but won't clear one that has already started.

Hot Baths or Sitz Baths: Temporary Relief Only

Soaking in warm water can soothe irritation, but it won't stop an infection from spreading.

- **Heat can temporarily ease discomfort but won't kill bacteria.**

- **Bathing incorrectly can worsen infections.** If bathwater is not clean, it can introduce new bacteria.

Avoiding Sexual Activity: Not a Practical Solution

Some people stop having sex entirely in an effort to prevent UTIs, but this is not a realistic or healthy approach.

- **Sexual activity is not the sole cause of UTIs.** Many people get UTIs without being sexually active, so abstinence isn't a guaranteed prevention method.

- **It ignores other contributing factors.** Hydration, diet, and microbiome health play a much bigger role in prevention than simply avoiding sex.

The Real Solution: A Comprehensive, Holistic Approach

If these common solutions don't work, what does? The key to breaking the cycle of recurrent UTIs lies in addressing the root causes rather than just treating symptoms. This means:

- Supporting **a balanced microbiome** in the gut, bladder, and vaginal tract.

- Strengthening **your immune system** through nutrition and lifestyle changes.

- Understanding **your personal triggers** and avoiding them.

- Managing stress and mental health, which can directly impact bladder health.

- Using a **proactive prevention plan** rather than reactive treatment.

Chapter 11

Creating Your Empowerment Plan – A Roadmap to Health and Healing

Urinary tract infections (UTIs) can feel like an endless cycle—one infection after another, leading to frustration, exhaustion, and a sense of powerlessness. But here's the truth: **you are not powerless.** You have the ability to take control of your health, break free from the cycle of recurrence, and reclaim your well-being. This chapter is about building your **Empowerment Plan**, a **personalized roadmap** to healing that takes your unique needs into account.

By the time you finish this chapter, you'll have a clear, actionable plan designed specifically for you. You'll understand **why past solutions failed,** what changes will make the biggest impact, and how to stay motivated on your path to long-term health.

This is where your healing truly begins.

Your Personalized Healing Plan

UTIs are often treated as **one-size-fits-all,** with antibiotics prescribed as the default solution. But healing isn't just about taking a pill—it's about addressing the root causes of your infections and **supporting your body's ability to heal and prevent future episodes.**

Creating a **Personalized Healing Plan** means taking a **holistic** approach, one that considers your unique body, triggers, and lifestyle. Below are the key elements of a **tailored plan** that works **for you, not just against the infection.**

Step 1: Identifying Your Triggers

The first step in breaking free from recurrent UTIs is understanding what's contributing to them. While bacteria are the direct cause, the conditions that allow bacteria to thrive vary from person to person. Ask yourself the following:

Lifestyle Triggers: Are certain activities (e.g., sex, holding in urine, dehydration) contributing to your UTIs?
Dietary Triggers: Are you consuming foods or drinks that irritate your urinary tract (e.g.,

caffeine, alcohol, artificial sweeteners)?
Hygiene & Habits: Are you using products
(e.g., scented soaps, harsh feminine washes)
that might be disrupting your vaginal flora?
Medical Triggers: Do you have underlying
conditions (e.g., hormonal imbalances,
diabetes, interstitial cystitis) that might be
making UTIs more frequent?

Use the **UTI Trigger Checklist** (included in the
workbook section) to help you identify patterns
and potential causes.

Step 2: Building Your Defense System

Once you know what's contributing to your
UTIs, it's time to **strengthen your body's
natural defenses.** Here's how:

1. Hydration & Urine pH Balance

- Drink at least **half your body weight in
  ounces** of water daily.

- Consider **alkalizing foods** (leafy greens,
  lemon water) to maintain an environment
  that discourages bacterial growth.

2. Bladder & Vaginal Microbiome Support

- Take **probiotics** (especially Lactobacillus species) to maintain a balanced vaginal flora.

- Eat fermented foods like **yogurt, sauerkraut, and kimchi** for natural probiotic support.

3. Strengthening the Immune System

- **Vitamin C, D, and Zinc** help your body fight infections more effectively.

- **Adequate sleep** and stress reduction are crucial for immune function.

4. Avoiding Irritants & Harmful Habits

- Switch to **fragrance-free, gentle personal care products.**

- Avoid tight synthetic clothing that **traps moisture** and creates a breeding ground for bacteria.

Step 3: Creating a Symptom Management & Prevention Toolkit

Your **Empowerment Plan** should include **both** short-term relief strategies and **long-term prevention** techniques.

Immediate Relief (Acute UTI Symptoms)

- **Hydrate aggressively** to flush bacteria.

- Use **herbal teas** (like marshmallow root and uva ursi) to soothe the bladder.

- Take **D-Mannose** if your UTIs are E. coli-related (but be aware it's not a cure-all).

- Use **heat packs** for temporary relief of pain and discomfort.

Long-Term Prevention

- **Pee after sex** and consider a **pH-balancing vaginal probiotic** if UTIs are sex-related.

- **Strengthen your bladder** with pelvic floor exercises like Kegels.

- **Balance vaginal health** by avoiding harsh cleansers and maintaining a healthy vaginal microbiome.

Breaking Free from the Cycle of Recurrence

One of the most frustrating aspects of recurrent UTIs is feeling like you're stuck in a never-ending cycle. You get an infection, take antibiotics, feel better for a while—then it happens all over again. **Why does this keep happening?**

The Root Cause Approach: Fixing the Foundation

To break free, you need to address **the underlying imbalances** that make you susceptible to frequent infections.

Key Strategies for Long-Term Healing

Restore Your Microbiome

- Frequent antibiotic use wipes out not only harmful bacteria but also **protective bacteria** that prevent infections.

- Consider **probiotic therapy** to replenish your beneficial bacteria and restore balance.

Support Your Body's Natural Defenses

- Your **immune system, vaginal health, and gut health** all play critical roles in preventing UTIs.

- Strengthening these areas **reduces reliance on medications** and helps your body fight infections naturally.

Address Underlying Conditions

- If you experience **hormonal changes, diabetes, or interstitial cystitis**, work with a practitioner to address these issues.

- Testing for **hidden infections or bladder dysfunctions** may reveal a deeper cause of recurrence.

Make Sustainable Lifestyle Adjustments

- **Hydration, diet, and stress management** play a huge role in UTI prevention.

- Implement small, sustainable changes that fit your lifestyle—this **isn't about perfection, it's about consistency.**

Staying Empowered on Your Path

Healing isn't always linear. Some days you'll feel **strong and symptom-free**, while others might bring setbacks. The key is to **stay committed** and know that every step you take is bringing you closer to lasting health.

Tools for Long-Term Success

Symptom & Trigger Tracking

- Keep a **UTI Journal** to track symptoms, triggers, and patterns.

- Note what worked and what didn't, so you can refine your approach.

Emotional Healing & Support

- The frustration, fear, and isolation of dealing with chronic UTIs are real.

- Join **support groups** (online or local) and connect with others who understand your journey.

Creating a Wellness Routine

- Integrate **daily self-care practices** (hydration, mindfulness, nutrition).

- Make prevention part of your lifestyle—not just a reaction to symptoms.

Final Words: You Are in Control

You've spent too much time feeling like UTIs dictate your life. But the truth is, **you have more control than you think.**

By creating your **Personalized Healing Plan**, breaking free from **recurrence cycles**, and staying **empowered with practical tools**, you can finally take back your health.

This is your journey. **And you are stronger than this condition.**

It's time to step into a future where **your body is resilient, your mind is confident, and your health is truly in your hands.**

Interactive Workbook Section

Your Empowerment Plan Worksheet (Fill in the blanks)

- My top **three triggers** are: _____

- The **key habits I need to change** are:

  _____

- My **daily prevention routine** will include:

  _____

- My **go-to strategies for symptom relief** are: _____

- My **long-term wellness goal** is:

  _____

Your Healing Journey Begins Now

A Final Note of Encouragement

Healing is not a straight path. It is a journey filled with twists, turns, setbacks, and breakthroughs. If you've made it to this point in the book, you've already taken one of the most important steps—you've empowered yourself with knowledge. That, in itself, is an act of reclaiming your health.

UTIs may have stolen your sense of control, your confidence in your body, and even your peace of mind. But today, you have a plan. You understand the root causes of recurrent infections, the limitations of common treatments, and the holistic strategies that will serve you for the long term. You are no longer at the mercy of yet another round of antibiotics, another painful night, or another dismissive doctor's visit.

Your journey doesn't end here. In fact, this is just the beginning. Healing is a daily commitment, a conscious choice to listen to your body, nurture it, and give it what it needs. Some days will be easier than others. There may still be moments of doubt or frustration, but now, you have tools to navigate them. You have the power to break free from the cycle of recurrence, the wisdom to prevent future infections, and the resilience to keep going, no matter what.

If you ever feel overwhelmed, remember that you are not alone. There is a whole community of people just like you who have been in your shoes—people who understand the struggle and have found their way to lasting relief. Stay connected, reach out for support, and keep learning. Every step forward, no matter how small, is a victory.

You deserve a life free from the pain and fear of UTIs. You deserve to wake up every day feeling strong, healthy, and in control of your body.

This is your journey. This is your healing. And it starts now.

Printed in Dunstable, United Kingdom